EPIDEMIC

CHRISTOPHER LAMPTON

THE MILLBROOK PRESS
BROOKFIELD, CT
A DISASTER! BOOK

Cover photograph courtesy of Peter Arnold, Inc.
Photographs courtesy of: Bettmann: pp. 6, 21, 41, 46–47 (both), 51; Bettmann/Hulton: p. 24;
Centers for Disease Control: pp. 8, 27, 45; World Health Organization: p. 10; Photo Researchers:
pp. 13, 28–29 (Biophoto Associates/Science Source), 33 (Hans Halberstadt), 39 (Dr. Arnold
Brody/Science Photo Library), 48 (Susan Kuklin), 53 (Will/Deni McIntyre); Culver Pictures: p. 17;
Historical Pictures Service: p. 18; National Library of Medicine: pp. 22, 23; Carolina Biological
Supply: pp. 37, 38; Magnum Photos (© Steele Perkins): p. 42.

Library of Congress Cataloging-in-Publication Data
Lampton, Christopher.
Epidemic / by Christopher Lampton.
p.   cm.—(A Disaster! book)
Includes bibliographical references and index.
Summary: Discusses how epidemics get started and spread, what can be done to prevent
them, and some of history's greatest, including the Black Death and AIDS.
ISBN 1-878841-92-0 (pbk.)
1. Epidemics—History—Juvenile literature. [1. Epidemics— History.] I. Title. II. Series:
Lampton, Christopher. Disaster! book.
RA643.L36   1992
614.4′9—dc20   91-21413 CIP AC

123456789 - WO - 96 95 94 93 92

CONTENTS

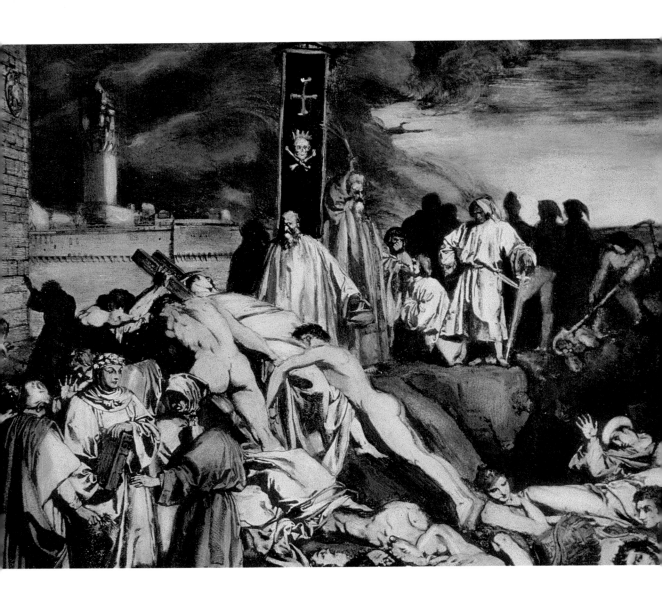

The Black Death in the city of Florence.

THE GREATEST DISASTER OF ALL

The greatest disaster in recorded history took place in the fourteenth century.

It began somewhere in Asia in the late 1330s. In 1347, it traveled to Europe by sea. Within the next four years, it killed more than 20 million people—one out of every three persons living in Europe at the time.

It was called the Black Death. Today we know it as the bubonic plague.

The bubonic plague is a disease caused by a tiny organism known as *Yersinia pestis.* It is often spread by the fleas that live on rats and bite humans. Some forms of the disease are spread among humans by coughing. The actual organism that causes plague is hurled into the air when the person coughs and is then breathed in by its next, unsuspecting victim.

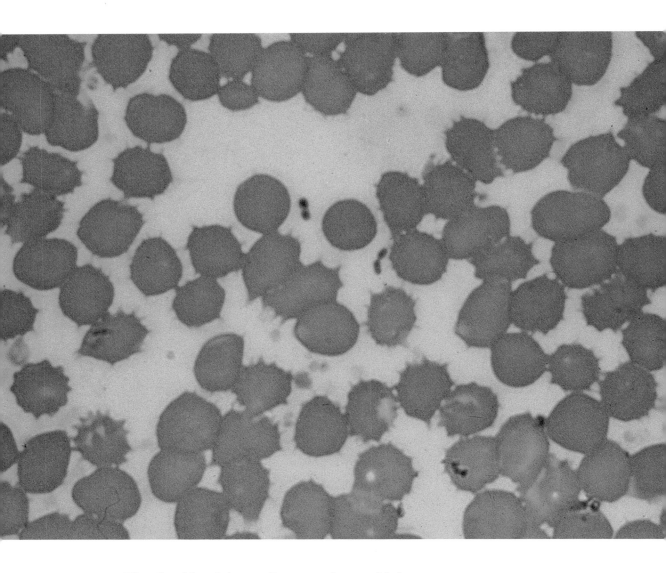

The tiny Yersinia pestis *organism, which lives on fleas that live on rats.*

But none of this was known in the fourteenth century. All that was really understood then about the disease was that it killed its victims within a few days—sometimes in a single evening—and that it was spreading like wildfire from place to place. The disease was so contagious that to be near someone who had it was almost a death sentence in itself. People lived in a constant panic, wondering who would be the next to die. They rarely had to wait long for the answer.

The Black Death probably began in central Asia, in part of what is today the Soviet Union. It was carried by the fleas that lived on a tiny animal called the marmot. Some natural disaster in the early fourteenth century must have killed off a lot of marmots, because the fleas moved from the marmots to rats. And the rats carried the fleas into the cities, where people live.

Ships traveling around the world often carry rats on board. Soon the disease had been carried by ship from Asia to Europe, the Middle East, and North Africa. And once the plague had taken hold in these places, there was no stopping it.

At times, entire shiploads of people would die before they could even reach port. Ghost ships, filled with the dead and dying, would drift ashore—passing on the disease to anyone who boarded the ship. And these people, in turn, would pass on the disease to other people that they met.

For the next four years, the Black Death moved across Europe, traveling from city to city and village to village. People would flee one town to escape the disease, only to find that they had carried the disease with them to another town.

No one was safe from the Black Death. It struck down old and young, weak and strong alike. But the poor were the hardest hit. They lived crammed together in close quarters, often among rats.

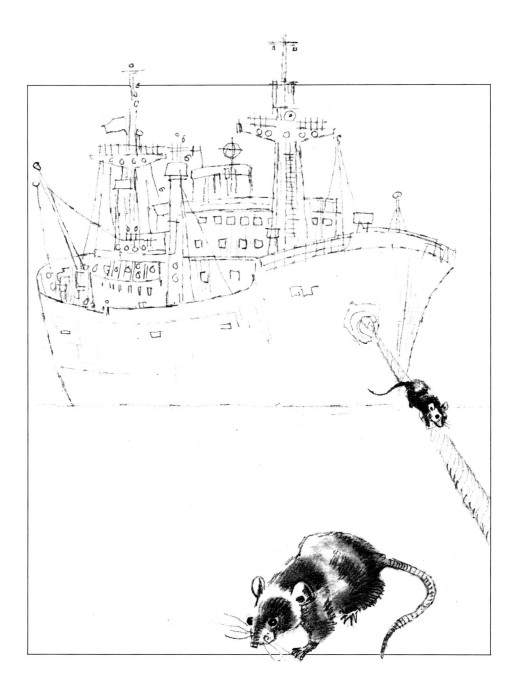

So swiftly did they die that their bodies would pile up in the streets, waiting for someone to carry them away to a mass grave.

Doctors were afraid to treat the sick and dying. They were afraid they might catch the disease themselves. It hardly mattered, though. The doctors weren't able to do much good. They had no idea how to treat the disease. In fact, many of the so-called "cures" for the disease, such as bloodletting, actually weakened the victims and made them more likely to die.

No one wanted to risk catching the plague. Priests fled from their congregations. Parents deserted their own children, and children ran away from their parents. Some people believed that the disease was a punishment from God, meant to eliminate all sinners from the human race. But sinners and saints alike were killed by the plague.

Just when it seemed that the world was coming to an end, the Black Death vanished. In 1351, four years after it had reached Europe, the disease burned itself out. But 20 million people in Europe and uncounted numbers elsewhere were dead. It was surely one of the most terrible disasters ever to befall the human race.

But it wasn't the only such disaster—not by a long shot.

Ships traveling around the world carrying rats spread many of the most famous plagues.

EPIDEMICS AND PANDEMICS

Diseases are always with us. On any given day, especially in the winter, you probably know of somebody who is home sick with a cold or "the flu." Sometimes, you or your friends may come down with even worse ailments, such as chicken pox or the measles. These are diseases that have been with the human race as far back as anybody was keeping records about such things. And it doesn't seem likely that they'll be disappearing any time in the near future. Fortunately, these are fairly mild diseases—at least in comparison with the Black Death.

Because these diseases are always with us, we say that they are *endemic.* This is a medical word that means "in the people." Doctors take it for granted that they will see a certain number of cases of the flu or measles every year, because these diseases are endemic to our society. Certainly, they are no cause for panic.

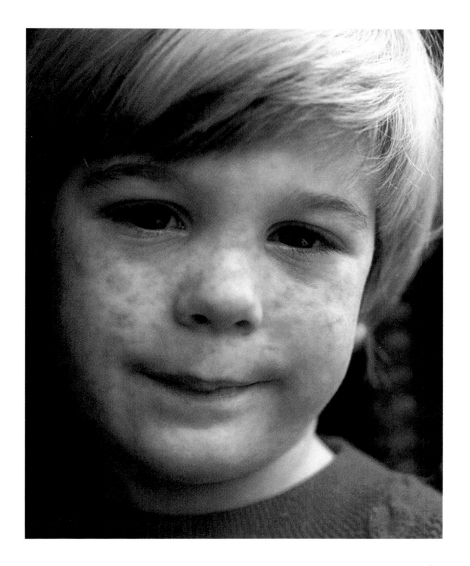

*Measles is still with us, in spite of massive
government programs to eradicate it.*

But every now and then a disease will begin to spread more rapidly than usual. An unexpectedly large number of cases will appear in doctors' offices. At that point, we say that there is an *epidemic* of the disease. Epidemic is a medical word that means "among the people." And when an epidemic spreads across much of the world, as the Black Death did, it is called a *pandemic,* meaning "all the people."

Although pandemics are fairly rare, epidemics happen all the time. They are most common in winter, when people spend a lot of time inside with other people. This makes it easier for diseases to spread from person to person. A typical epidemic will last for a few weeks before the disease returns to its normal levels.

Most epidemics are not disastrous. A few people may die of the disease, but the majority get sick for a few days and then recover. Some epidemics, however, are more severe than others. And every now and then an epidemic will get out of hand and become a pandemic. Large numbers of people may die, as happened with the Black Death.

Although we think of great pandemics as something out of the distant past, the last one actually occurred in the twentieth century, during the first world war. And there may be more great pandemics in store for us in the future. Some scientists think that the disease AIDS could become the next major pandemic. Furthermore, there are large epidemics currently raging through the poorer countries of the world, where diseases cannot be fought as effectively as in the wealthier nations. Although these are not pandemics, because they take place only within certain countries, they nonetheless affect a large portion of the world's population.

Epidemiologists (EP-eh-dee-mee-OL-oh-jists) are scientists who study epidemics. They try to determine who in society at large is likely to get the disease, how they will get it, how many people will get sick each year, and so forth. The term *epidemic* is often used to describe any illness that is more common than usual. This includes heart disease and cancer. But in this book we are going to talk only about epidemics of so-called *communicable diseases*. These are diseases that are *contagious*—that is, that are spread by people.

Later, we'll talk about the causes and cures of these communicable diseases. But first, let's look at a few more of the great epidemics and pandemics of ages past.

EPIDEMICS THROUGHOUT HISTORY

■ *The Plague of Athens.* There have probably been epidemics and pandemics as long as there have been human beings—longer, if you count epidemics among other species. But the first great pandemic in recorded history took place nearly 2,500 years ago, in ancient Athens.

The plague struck Athens in the year 430 B.C. This was during the Peloponnesian Wars, when Athens was at war with neighboring Sparta. When the troops came home for the winter, a mysterious disease seemed to follow them, though nobody is sure where it came from. It probably started in Ethiopia and had already visited Egypt, Libya, and Persia (now Iran) before it reached Athens.

At first, people came down with a mild fever that lasted for a few days and was gone. But then the disease became deadly. After seven or eight days, most of the new victims died. Even those who

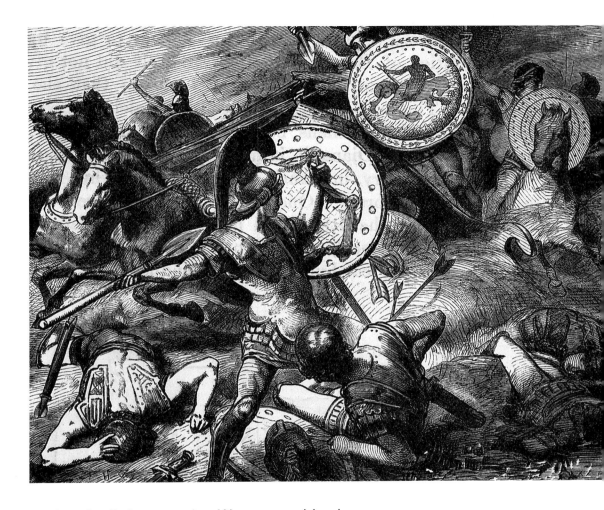

*During the Peloponnesian Wars, an epidemic
struck down much of the Greek population.
Invading armies often unknowingly spread
deadly communicable diseases, sometimes
causing more harm than the war itself.*

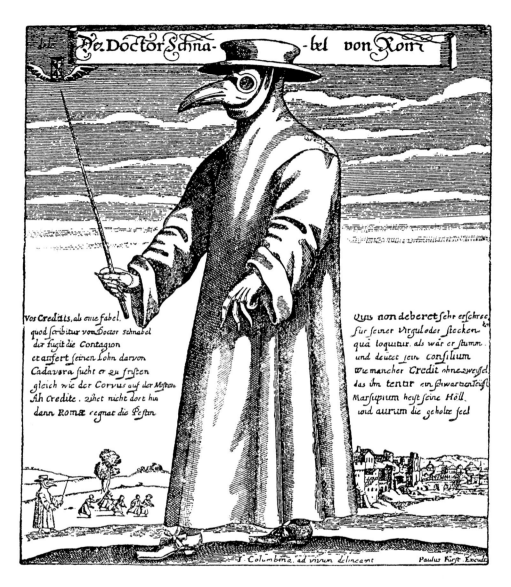

A plague doctor in clothing designed to protect from contagion.

survived often lost the use of their fingers, toes, or other organs. Some became amnesiacs, unable to remember their own names.

At that time there were no medicines that could relieve the suffering. The epidemic lasted for four years before finally vanishing. To this day, no one is quite sure what disease the Athenians had. It may have been the bubonic plague, smallpox, measles, scarlet fever, or even the flu. But nobody really knows.

■ *The Great Plague of Constantinople.* The bubonic plague has returned again and again to ravage humanity. The disease is never completely gone. The *Yersinia pestis* organism lives on the fleas carried by rats and other small animals. Even when no human being is suffering from bubonic plague, it lies in wait, ready to strike again.

The first recorded outbreak of bubonic plague among human beings was in A.D. 541. (At least, this is the first epidemic that we *know* to be bubonic plague. It's possible that earlier epidemics, such as the plague of Athens, were also bubonic plague.) The outbreak occurred in the mighty Byzantine Empire, and by the year 542 the plague had reached Constantinople, home of the emperor Justinian. At its height, ten thousand people a day were dying from the disease. Even the emperor himself was taken sick, though he apparently survived. By the end of the year, however, the disease was fading. It would not return again in force until the Black Death of the fourteenth century.

■ *The Great Plague of London.* The last major epidemic of the bubonic plague struck England in 1665. In fact, it had never entirely gone away after the Black Death three centuries earlier. But suddenly it came back in force, mostly in the slums of London, where people lived huddled together in filthy, rat-infested housing. The worst attack of the disease came during an unusually hot summer. Large portions of the city were quarantined (isolated) in an attempt to keep the disease from spreading. More than two thousand people a week died in London that summer, with over seven thousand dying during a single week in September. By late fall, the disease began to fade. And by the end of the year, it was gone.

It never returned. Many people believed that it had been chased away by the Great Fire of London in 1666. But there's no medical basis for this belief. More likely, changes in the rat population of London altered the way in which the disease was spread.

■ *The cholera epidemics of the nineteenth century.* The disease known as cholera has long been endemic to much of Asia, particularly around India. But in the early nineteenth century, it suddenly began to spread to the rest of the world, including China, Japan, the Middle East, and eventually England. By 1832, it even reached the United States, killing thousands of people from New York to New Orleans.

Cholera usually begins with diarrhea that is very watery. Vomiting sometimes accompanies the diarrhea. Victims rapidly become weaker and weaker, until they go into shock. Death then follows.

Nobody knew what caused cholera or how to prevent it. Then a doctor named John Snow performed a clever experiment. It was from that experiment that modern epidemiology was born.

Snow noticed in 1854 that most of the people in London who were dying of cholera were drinking water from a single pump located at the corner of Broad Street and Cambridge. He analyzed the water from the pump and discovered that it contained strange white particles. These particles were just like particles he had seen in the diarrhea of people with the disease. Somehow the pump water

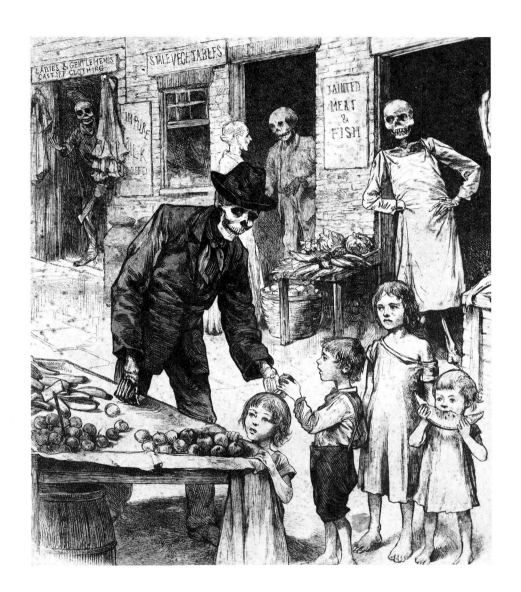

Unsanitary conditions contribute to many epidemics.

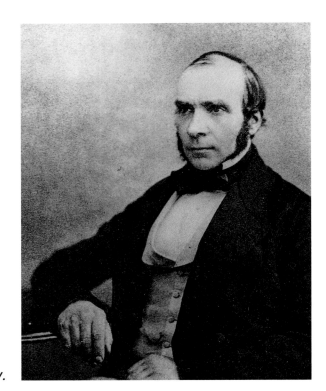

Dr. John Snow, discoverer of the cause of the cholera epidemic of London in the 1850s. Snow is also the father of modern epidemiology.

was becoming contaminated with sewage. It was spreading the disease to everyone who drank from it. When Snow convinced city officials to shut down the pump, the disease almost vanished from London.

Once it was realized that the disease came from drinking contaminated water, it was possible to prevent its spread. Cholera has almost ceased to exist in those countries that can afford to keep their water supplies sanitary, or clean. But in the poorer countries of the world, unsanitary conditions still exist. Cholera remains endemic to these areas.

■ *The Spanish flu of 1918.* Pandemics often take place during war. This is because moving armies carry diseases with them to distant corners of the world. The Spanish flu of 1918 broke out during the final year of World War I and spread across the world with remarkable speed. Epidemiologists regard it as one of the three greatest epidemics of recorded history, along with the Great Plague of Constantinople and the Black Death.

INFLUENZA

FREQUENTLY COMPLICATED WITH

PNEUMONIA

IS PREVALENT AT THIS TIME THROUGHOUT AMERICA.

THIS THEATRE IS CO-OPERATING WITH THE DEPARTMENT OF HEALTH.

YOU MUST DO THE SAME

IF YOU HAVE A COLD AND ARE COUGHING AND SNEEZING. DO NOT ENTER THIS THEATRE

GO HOME AND GO TO BED UNTIL YOU ARE WELL

Coughing, Sneezing or Spitting Will Not Be Permitted In The Theatre. In case you must cough or Sneeze, do so in your own hand- kerchief, and if the Coughing or Sneezing Persists Leave The Theatre At Once.

This Theatre has agreed to co-operate with the Department Of Health in disseminating the truth about Influenza, and thus serve a great educational purpose.

HELP US TO KEEP CHICAGO THE HEALTHIEST CITY IN THE WORLD

JOHN DILL ROBERTSON

COMMISSIONER OF HEALTH

A 1918 influenza poster issued by the Chicago Commissioner of Health.

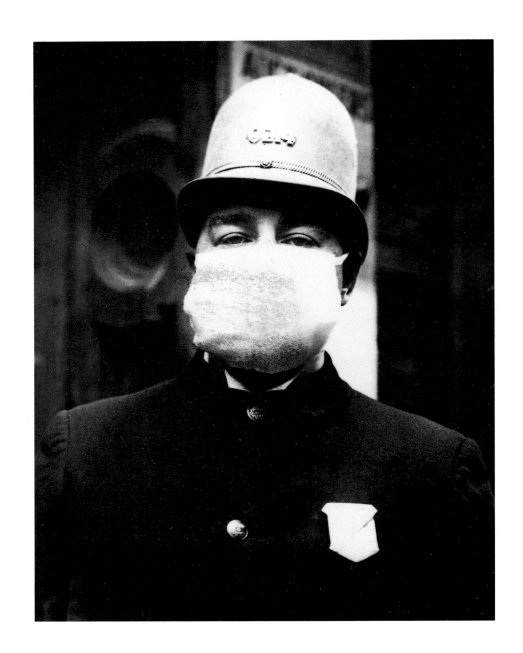

24

The disease seems to have begun at an army post in Kansas. From there it spread to Europe as divisions of soldiers were sent away to battle. However, people at the time for some reason thought that it had started in Spain, so the disease became known popularly as the Spanish influenza. Starting in the spring of 1918, it spread around the world. By fall, it had already become one of the worst epidemics of all time.

The epidemic was probably started by what is today called type-A influenza. The number of deaths it caused was staggering. In one week in October of 1918, 21,000 people died in the United States alone. By the time the epidemic finally came to an end in the spring of 1919, more than 20 million people had died worldwide. Unlike most other communicable diseases, which often kill only the very young and the very old, the Spanish flu killed people of all ages, striking down millions of people in the prime of their lives.

Could the disease come back again? It's possible. And, as we'll see later in this book, some experts believed that it was going to return in the year 1976. But, even if it does return, medicines are now available that would greatly lessen the impact of the epidemic. It's unlikely that another flu epidemic could occur that would be as devastating as the one in 1918.

An American policeman shows his flu mask during the influenza epidemic of 1918–1919.

WHAT CAUSES DISEASE?

All communicable diseases are caused by tiny organisms, much too small to see. These organisms can take up residence in the human body. Once there, they can multiply, often harming or even destroying part of the body.

The human body, of course, fights back against this invasion. The battle between our bodies and the tiny invading organisms is what we call sickness or disease. It can produce symptoms ranging from fever to stomachaches and headaches. It can eventually result in death.

These tiny organisms often move from one person to another. When this happens, we say that the disease is *contagious,* or "catching." Different organisms spread in different ways. The organisms that cause the flu and colds, for instance, are spread by hand-to-mouth contact. The organisms that cause malaria and yellow fever are spread by mosquito bites.

Doctors refer to these tiny disease-causing organisms as *pathogens.* The most common types of pathogens are *viruses, bacteria,* and *fungi.* Viruses are so small and simple that scientists debate whether they should actually be considered living organisms. They consist of a small shell made out of protein. This shell contains a long strand of a substance known as *nucleic acid. Deoxyribonucleic acid,* or *DNA* for short, is the main nucleic acid. (A few viruses contain a strand of a similar substance called *ribonucleic acid,* or *RNA* for short.)

This photograph shows the AIDS virus, HIV-1 (the small, round particles), amid the body's T lymphocytes. T lymphocytes are a kind of white blood cell used to fight infection.

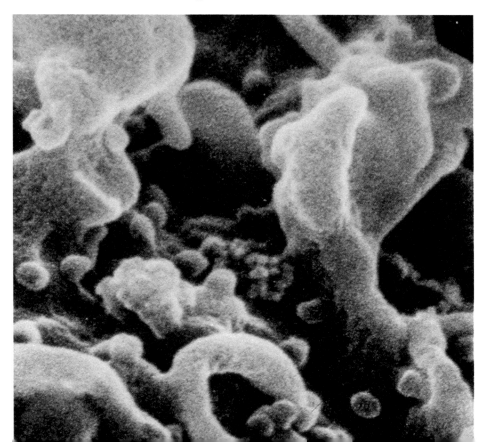

All living creatures, including humans, are made out of tiny components called *cells*. These cells are the basic building blocks of life. Like viruses, the cells of all living creatures contain DNA and RNA.

There are many different kinds of cells in our bodies. Our skin is made up of skin cells, our muscles are made up of specialized

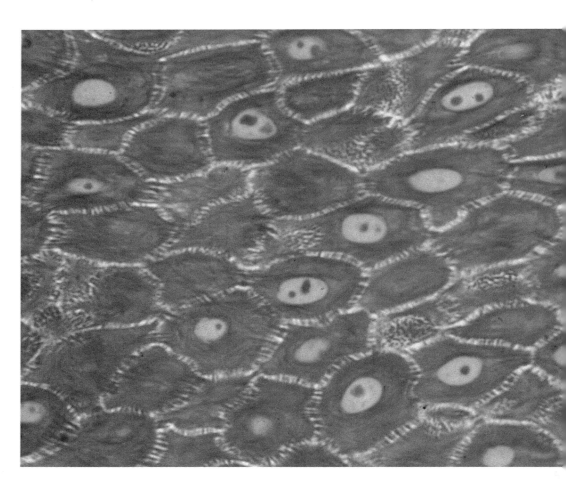

muscle cells, our brains are made up of cells called neurons, and so forth. These cells are much too small to see with the naked eye, but we are made up of trillions of them.

Viruses can't grow or multiply on their own. They must attach themselves to living cells. Once attached, the viruses—like miniature hypodermic needles—inject their strands of DNA into the cell.

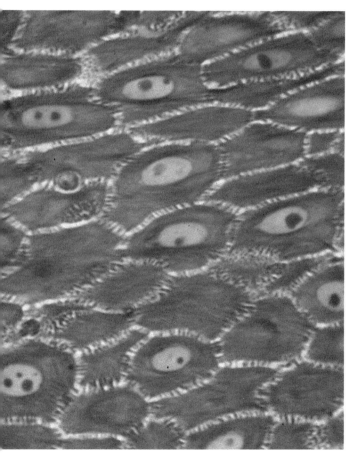

Skin cells are only one of the many different kinds of cells in our bodies.

These strands of DNA contain instructions, written in a language called the *genetic code.* The instructions are for manufacturing the proteins and nucleic acids that are needed to build more viruses. The cell is forced to put aside its own set of instructions for cell building and follow these. Viruses by the thousands are produced. So many copies of the viruses are made that the cell eventually fills up and bursts open. Thousands of new viruses escape into the body, where each can invade and destroy still more cells. This is how viruses cause disease.

Because different types of viruses attack different types of cells, they cause different types of disease. Diseases caused by viruses include smallpox, rabies, polio, yellow fever, measles, and AIDS.

Bacteria are larger than viruses. And they are definitely living organisms, each made up of a single cell. Many bacteria live harmlessly in the bodies of animals, without causing disease. The human intestines, for instance, contain roughly a pound of bacteria. These bacteria help us to digest food. But other types of bacteria manufacture poisonous substances that can make us ill. Diseases caused by bacteria include cholera, typhoid fever, tetanus, and bubonic plague.

Fungi are a type of plant and usually don't cause disease. Mushrooms, for instance, are a type of non–disease-causing fungus (singular of *fungi*). Some varieties of mushroom, however, are poisonous. Also, some fungi live on the human body and cause annoying but generally not serious conditions such as athlete's foot and ringworm, as well as a few deadly but rare diseases.

Some diseases are caused by *parasites.* These are actually tiny animals, some as small as a single cell, others as large as insects. Parasites take up residence in the bodies of human beings and other animals. Often, they make the person whose body they reside in quite ill. They can be spread in food, water, and even in the bodies of insects such as mosquitoes. Diseases caused by parasites include malaria and trypanosomiasis (sleeping sickness). Parasitic diseases are most common in countries in the tropics, near the equator.

CURING
ILLNESS

Until the end of the nineteenth century, there was little that doctors could do for victims of a contagious disease. A doctor's task was simply to make patients as comfortable as possible until they either got better on their own or died.

Then, in the nineteenth century, doctors finally came to understand how pathogens spread from person to person. They learned to take precautions against contagious disease. Surgeons began scrubbing their hands before surgery in order to remove disease-causing organisms. They saved countless lives in the process. Hospital equipment was *sterilized* (made free of pathogens, usually by heating). Wounds were cleaned. Suddenly, the number of people who survived medical emergencies began to climb.

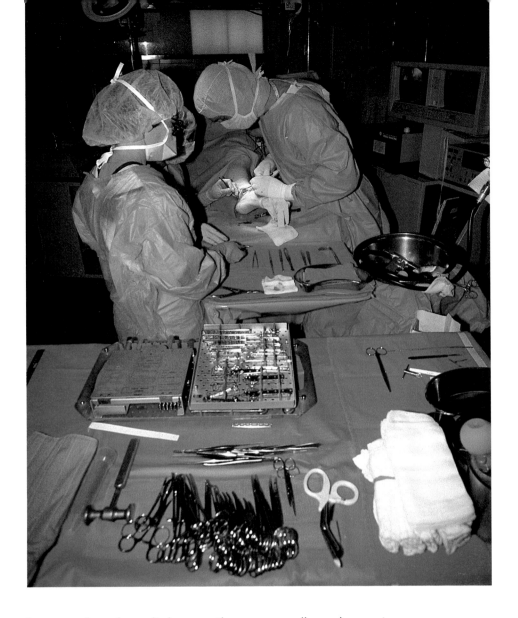

In a modern hospital operating room, all equipment
and clothing is sterilized so as not to spread disease.
This has saved countless lives.

In fact, improved sanitation procedures are one of the most important weapons in the war against epidemic diseases. We saw earlier how Dr. Snow stopped a cholera epidemic in London by shutting down a single, unsanitary pump. Similarly, large-scale sanitation procedures, such as sterilization of milk and purification of water, have put an end to many epidemic diseases of centuries past. The extermination (mass killing) of insects and rodents that carry disease has also been an important factor in fighting epidemics.

In the twentieth century, doctors have a large arsenal of medicines that can be used to cure disease. A few of these medicines were actually available in centuries past as folk remedies. But doctors had largely dismissed the folk remedies' ability to cure.

Probably the most famous of these modern "miracle drugs" are the *antibiotics.* These are chemicals, such as penicillin, that are able to kill or prevent the multiplication of an invading bacterium (singular of *bacteria*). In many cases, these chemicals are produced in nature by the pathogens themselves in their continuing war with other pathogens. Penicillin, for instance, is produced by a type of fungus. Because antibiotics are harmless to most human beings but harmful to bacteria, they can cure the disease without harming the patient. If antibiotics had been available in centuries past, many of the great epidemics of history, such as the Black Death, would never have happened.

Antibiotics aren't effective against viruses and fungi. Fortunately, medical science has begun to develop antiviral and antifungal agents that can fight even these pathogens. Antiviral agents, for instance, often take the form of certain chemicals. These chemicals can destroy the strands of DNA injected into cells by viruses before the cell begins to build new copies of the virus.

There's an old saying that an ounce of prevention is worth a pound of cure. And one of the best ways of fighting a disease is to keep it from happening in the first place. To do that, doctors have learned to work with the oldest disease-fighting system of all—the one inside your body.

THE IMMUNE SYSTEM

Not all diseases can be cured by medicine. Fortunately, the human body has its own defenses for fighting viruses and other pathogenic invaders. This group of defenses is known as the *immune system.*

A large part of our bodies' defense against foreign invaders is the human skin. Skin provides a kind of wall between the working machinery of the body and the world outside. This wall can keep pathogens out. Alas, pathogens can still enter the body through openings such as the nose and mouth. But even here there are traps and barriers to catch pathogens before they can do damage. The nose, for instance, contains tiny hairs and maze-like passages to trap any unwanted organisms that try to enter through it.

If a pathogen manages to get past all of these barriers, the most impressive part of the immune system comes into play. Ex-

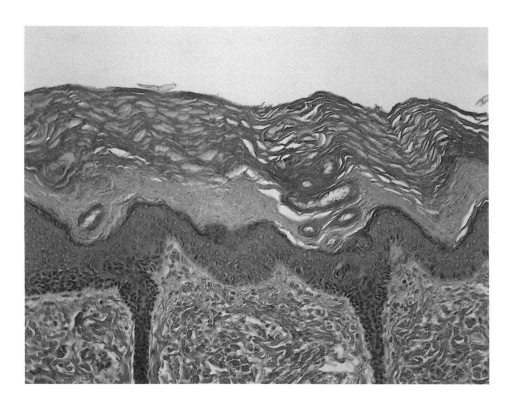

*Human skin forms a very effective
barrier against invading organisms.*

tremely tiny cellular "machines" inside the body can seek out and
destroy the invaders, like antiballistic missiles repelling an incoming
warhead. The most important of these are the *leukocytes,* or *white
blood cells.* Leukocytes perform a number of different tasks in the
war against invading pathogens. A type of leukocyte called a *macrophage* can actually surround a pathogen and "eat" it.

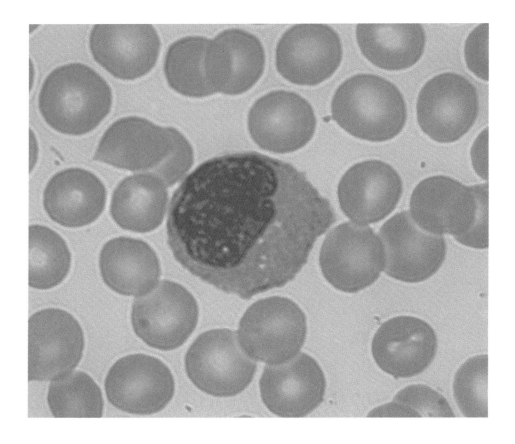

Above: White blood cells are the soldiers that defend the body's organs against tiny invaders. Right: Two macrophages at work in a human lung. In this picture, taken with a camera attached to a scanning electron microscope, the top macrophage is its normal rounded shape. But the one below has elongated itself to engulf the small particle at left—perhaps a piece of dust or pollen.

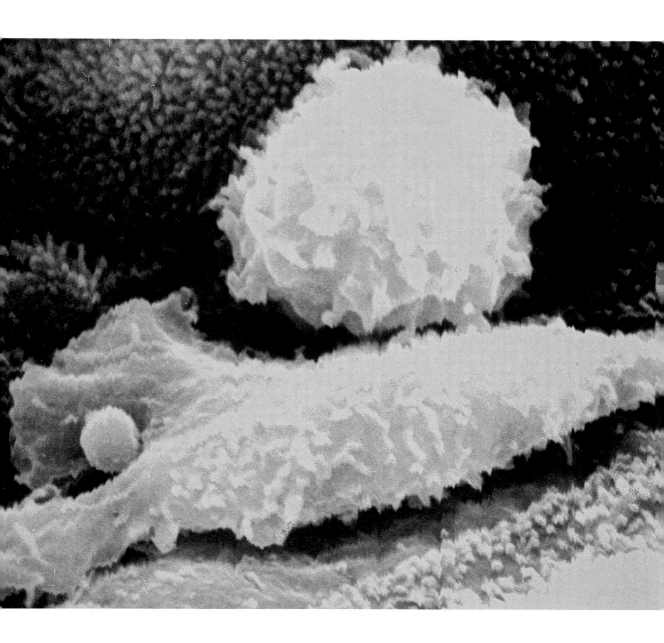

39

In response to an attack by pathogens, the body's leukocytes help design special proteins called *antibodies.* These recognize specific pathogens by their shape. These antibodies attach themselves to structures called *antigens* on the surface of the pathogens. They kill the pathogens and then eliminate them from the body. Even after you've recovered from a disease, the antibodies will remain. They can recognize the same pathogen should it attack a second time and put it out of commission before it can do any harm. This is why people often become *immune* to a disease after they have had it a single time.

The immune system doesn't always chase away a pathogen in time to save the life of a victim. Thus, some forms of medical treatment involve giving the body a head start against pathogens. Doctors can inject weakened or killed forms of a pathogen into a patient's body. This allows the immune system to form antibodies against the pathogen and respond appropriately should the patient be exposed to the real thing. These injections are called *vaccines.*

Some vaccines are made up of actual living pathogens that have been made too weak to cause disease. These are called *live vaccines.* Others are made of dead viruses. These are called *killed vaccines.* The main drawback to live-virus vaccines is that, in a few rare cases, they can cause the disease that they are meant to prevent. But they also produce a much more powerful immunity to disease than do killed-virus vaccines.

Physicians can inject vaccines directly into the bloodstream. Patients, however, do not always immediately appreciate the medical benefits.

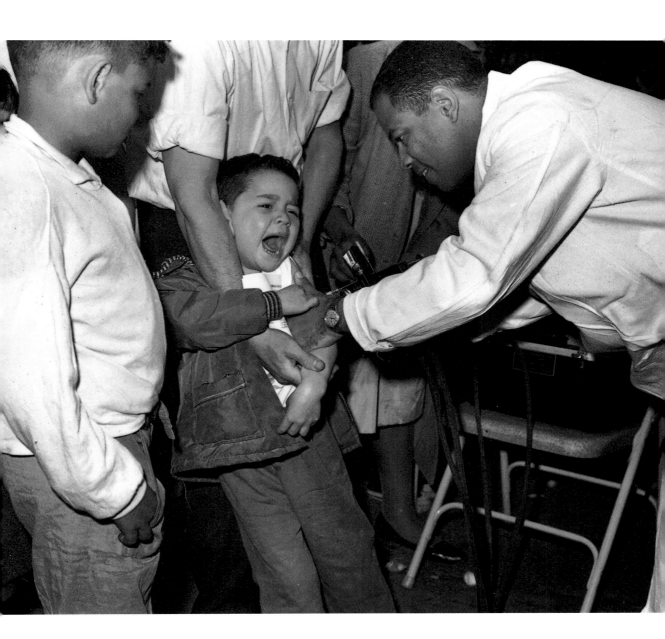

41

The most frightening communicable diseases today are those, such as AIDS, that not only fail to respond to medicine but can avoid the immune system as well. In fact, AIDS (which is short for acquired immune deficiency syndrome) actually destroys the immune system of the victim.

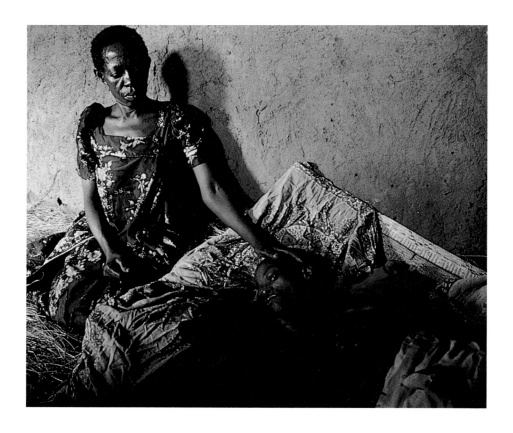

AIDS in Africa is already a raging epidemic, claiming thousands of lives, young and old, men and women.

TYPES OF EPIDEMIC DISEASES

There are thousands of different diseases to which human beings can fall victim. Many of these are communicable—that is, they can be spread from person to person. Here are some of the best known:

■ *Influenza.* Also known as the flu, this is one of the most common of epidemic diseases. It is extremely contagious. The symptoms resemble those of a severe cold. The flu is often a relatively mild illness. But it can lead to pneumonia, bronchitis, and death. Major flu epidemics occur every decade or so. However, they are rarely as bad as the Spanish flu epidemic of 1918 that we discussed earlier in this book.

■ *Smallpox.* At one time smallpox was one of the most feared of epidemic diseases. It practically ceased to exist in the late 1970s as a result of an international campaign to eliminate it from the world population. The only remaining smallpox viruses in the world today are kept in two laboratories for research purposes. The last known case of smallpox occurred in 1979 when a laboratory worker was accidentally exposed to the virus. Two years earlier, the last naturally occurring case was recorded. The disease gets its name from the pockmarks that it leaves on the skin. Survivors of smallpox were often left permanently scarred by these marks.

■ *Bubonic plague.* It may not be very common anymore, but bubonic plague is probably the most famous of the great epidemic diseases. Its symptoms include a high fever and chills. But the symptom that gives the disease its name is the appearance of buboes, or large swollen bumps, on the body of the victim. There are two forms of the disease. The other, known as pneumonic plague, infects the lungs and spreads its pathogens through the air every time the victim breathes out or coughs. This is the most contagious form of the disease and also the most deadly. It almost always kills its victims within three days if not treated. Fortunately, there are antibiotics available today that can stop the disease in its tracks, but in the Middle Ages it was incurable. Because the bacterium that causes the disease lives on the fleas of certain rats, epidemics of plague would often occur whenever a city or country decided to exterminate its rat population. The fleas, having no more rats to live on, would begin to bite human beings and give them the disease.

■ *Yellow fever.* This disease of the tropics takes its name from the jaundiced, or yellowish, color of the victim's skin. Symptoms include fever, internal bleeding, nausea, and headaches. Death often results. Yellow fever was once a major killer in South and Central

America, and there have even been outbreaks in the southern United States. Modern vaccination techniques, however, have reduced outbreaks to occasional minor epidemics. Yellow fever is caused by a virus that lives in mosquitoes. It is usually spread from person to person through the bite of these infected mosquitoes.

Yellow fever is spread from person to person through the bite of infected mosquitoes.

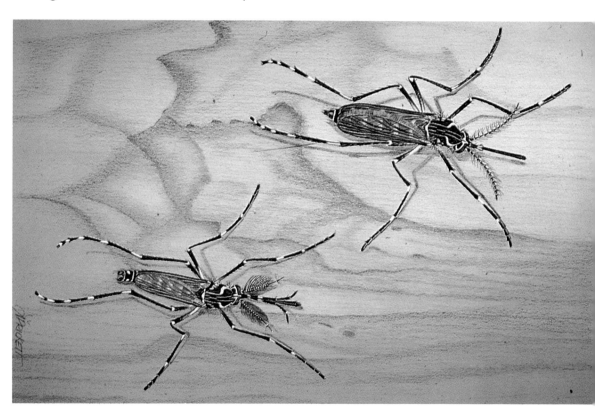

■ *Poliomyelitis.* Mild cases of polio (as the disease is more commonly known) cause only slight fever and weakness. However, the virus can sometimes enter the victim's nervous system and leave him or her paralyzed for life. During the great polio epidemics of the

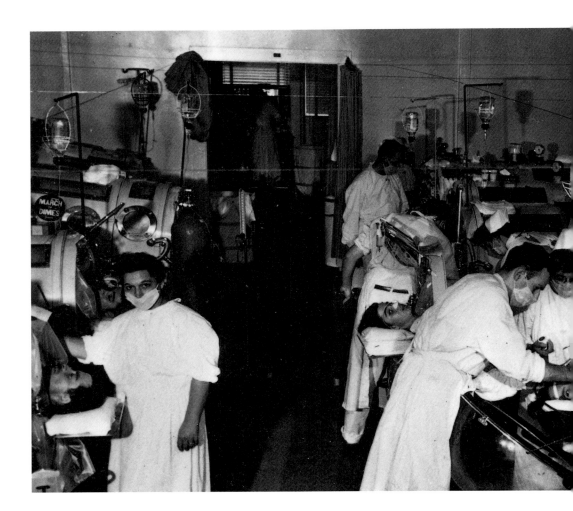

1940s and 1950s, thousands of children (and many older people) lost the use of their legs or arms. Sometimes the muscles involved in breathing were also paralyzed. Fortunately, a killed-virus polio vaccine was developed in 1953 by Dr. Jonas Salk. (It was later

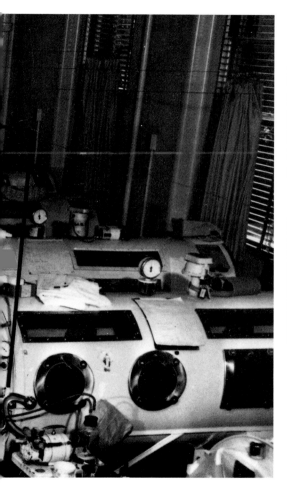

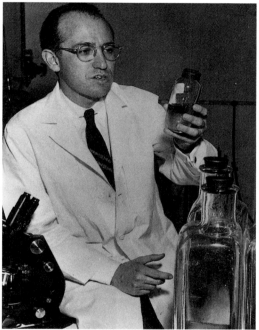

Above: Dr. Jonas Salk, inventor of the killed-virus polio vaccine. Left: The severe polio epidemics of the 1940s and 50s caused thousands of young Americans to require these iron lungs in order to breathe.

replaced by a live-virus vaccine developed by Dr. Alfred Sabin.) The disease is now relatively rare, but it is still important for children to receive polio vaccinations. Without the vaccinations, new epidemics of polio could still occur.

The Sabin vaccine is usually given orally, or by mouth.

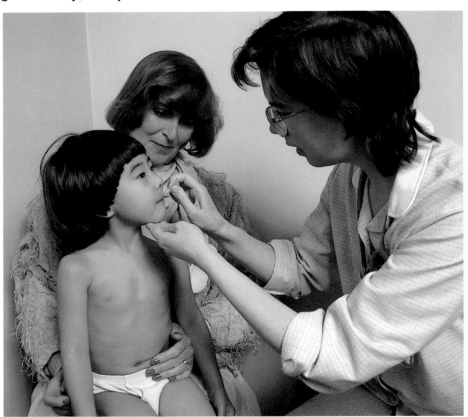

PREDICTING EPIDEMICS

There are now vaccines available for hundreds or even thousands of epidemic diseases. (In many cases, there are several vaccines for a single type of disease. This is necessary because the pathogens that cause the disease can come in several different *strains,* or types. Different strains sometimes require separate vaccinations, although frequently the vaccinations for several strains are mixed together in a single injection.) Young children are generally vaccinated against the most devastating and common diseases, such as polio.

It would be useful if doctors and scientists could predict in advance when an epidemic is going to strike. That way, all of those at risk for that disease could be vaccinated a few months before the epidemic was due to arrive. The epidemic might never take place.

Is it possible to predict an epidemic in advance? Yes and no.

There are patterns in the way that epidemics occur. But successfully predicting the exact strain of the disease, not to mention exactly when the epidemic will arrive, is tricky indeed. Epidemics of the flu, for instance, generally occur every decade or so. But they rarely occur right on schedule.

In 1976, doctors attempted to predict the arrival of an epidemic—and failed. Many doctors believed that the strain of flu that caused the devastating pandemic in 1918, now known as swine flu because it can also infect pigs, was going to return. The 1918 pandemic was one of the most severe in history, and nobody wanted it to happen again. The president of the United States, then Gerald Ford, announced that mass vaccinations would be given free to the American public to prevent the epidemic.

But the vaccinations weren't very popular. Few people showed up for them, and the epidemic still didn't happen. Doctors had jumped the gun on their prediction, though they had good medical reasons for believing that the epidemic was going to happen. The science of predicting epidemics is still very imperfect.

Once an epidemic has begun, it is possible to make predictions about the course it will take. There are even computer programs that can "model" the progress of the epidemic. These programs are based on the idea that epidemics occur when each victim of the disease, on average, passes on the disease to more than one other person. That way, the number of people suffering from the disease increases rapidly—which is the very definition of an epidemic.

Eventually, there are enough people who have had the disease and are immune to it. The victims can no longer pass it on to enough other people to sustain the epidemic. The epidemic gradually comes to an end, even though there are still quite a few people in the population who haven't had the disease. When enough people in a

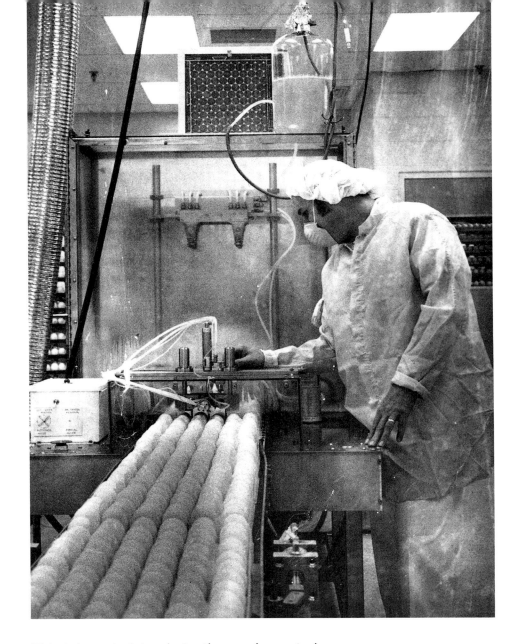

*This lab technician is testing various strains
of the swine flu virus with the new vaccine.*

population are immune to a disease that an epidemic can no longer take hold, we say that that population of people has *herd immunity*. (This term was probably first used by epidemiologists studying epidemic diseases in populations of animals, such as cows.)

It is important for epidemiologists to predict the point at which herd immunity will stop an epidemic. This helps them to determine how many people must be vaccinated against the disease in order to stop it. It's not possible to vaccinate everyone against a disease. But it's only necessary to vaccinate enough people for herd immunity to take effect.

Parents don't pass on their immunity to a disease to their children. So, as a new generation grows up, herd immunity is lost. Eventually, there are many, many people in the population who are not immune to the disease. Then the epidemic can return and strike the population once again.

Perhaps the most frustrating thing about epidemic diseases to a doctor is that they keep changing. Even as human beings are developing new ways to cure diseases, the diseases are developing new ways to avoid being cured. Many diseases eventually become resistant to the medicines used to fight them. This means that the pathogen causing a disease becomes altered genetically and is now able to resist, or fight, the medicine. When this happens, that medicine is no longer effective in treating the disease.

A researcher, wearing protective clothing and working under a protective hood, studies the deadly AIDS virus.

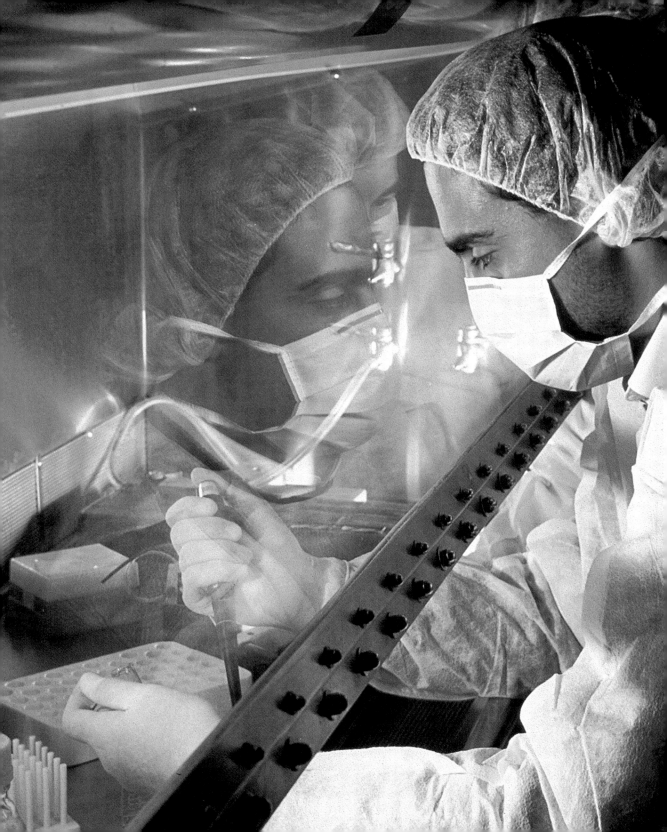

Malaria, for instance, is a disease endemic to the tropics. It has been successfully fought with medicines for many years. Now the pathogen that causes malaria is starting to become resistant to those medicines, and epidemics of malaria are starting to recur. This is happening with other diseases as well.

The war between human beings and pathogens will probably continue for a long time to come. Doctors and scientists have learned a lot in recent years about treating diseases. But nature still has a few tricks left up its sleeve!

GLOSSARY

antibiotics—chemicals that doctors prescribe to kill or prevent the spread of invading bacteria.

antibodies—special proteins made by white blood cells. Antibodies recognize pathogens and prevent them from re-entering the body to cause disease again.

antigens—structures on the surface of pathogens to which antibodies can attach themselves.

bacterium (pl., *bacteria*)—a small organism consisting of a single cell that can invade the body of a human being or other living organism and cause disease.

cell—one of the tiny components of which all living organisms are made.

communicable disease—a disease that can be spread from one individual to another by the passing on of tiny organisms known as pathogens.

contagious—refers to a disease that is communicable, that is, one that can be spread from individual to individual.

deoxyribonucleic acid (DNA)—a substance contained within the cells of all living organisms, as well as the protein shells of viruses. It contains instructions for assembling new copies of that organism (or virus).

endemic—from Greek words meaning "in the people," describes a disease that is always present in a population.

epidemic—from Greek words meaning "among the people," describes a disease that is present in a population in more than its usual numbers.

epidemiologist—a scientist who studies the patterns of disease in a population, that is, how it spreads and whom it attacks.

fungus (pl., *fungi*)—a type of plant that can cause disease.

genetic code—the "language" in which information is written on strands of DNA.

herd immunity—the immunity of a population to a disease, even when some individuals in the population are not immune.

immune system—the defense system in the human body (and the bodies of other living organisms) that repels pathogens that invade the body and cause disease.

killed vaccine—a vaccine made up of dead pathogens or fragments of pathogens.

leukocytes—also known as white blood cells, these disease-fighting cells can be divided into five types that serve different roles in the immune system to fight invading pathogens.

live vaccine—a vaccine made up of actual living, but weakened, pathogens.

macrophage—a special type of cell used by the human immune system to "eat" invading pathogens.

nucleic acid—a substance found in living cells and in viruses; nucleic acids come in two varieties, ribonucleic acid (RNA) and deoxyribonucleic acid (DNA).

pandemic—from Greek words meaning "all the people," describes an epidemic disease that has spread over much of the world.

parasite—a tiny animal that lives in or on the body of another living creature and can cause disease.

pathogen—a tiny organism, such as a virus or bacterium, that can invade the body of another organism, such as a human being, and cause disease.

ribonucleic acid (RNA)—a substance similar to deoxyribonucleic acid (DNA).

sterilize—to make free of disease-causing pathogens, usually by heating or chemical means.

strain—a specific form of a pathogen, such as a virus or a bacterium. Some pathogens come in several different strains. Immunity to one strain does not necessarily mean immunity to others.

vaccine—an injection consisting of a killed or weakened form of a pathogen. Vaccines allow the immune system to create antibodies that will recognize that pathogen and prevent it from causing disease in the future.

virus—an extremely small pathogen that consists of a shell made out of protein. Viruses contain tightly coiled strands of DNA or RNA, which can be injected into a living cell. The DNA then causes the cell to produce new copies of the virus. This eventually destroys the cell and causes disease.

white blood cells—see *leukocytes*.

Yersinia pestis—the bacterium that causes bubonic plague.

RECOMMENDED READING

Knight, David C. *Viruses—Life's Smallest Enemies.* New York: William Morrow & Co., 1981.

——————. *Your Body's Defenses.* New York: McGraw-Hill, 1975.

LeMaster, Leslie Jean. *Bacteria and Viruses.* Chicago: Childrens Press, 1985.

Nourse, Alan E. *Your Immune System.* New York: Franklin Watts, 1989.

INDEX

ABOUT THE AUTHOR

Christopher Lampton is a free-lance writer. Born in Brownsville, Texas, he has a bachelor of arts degree in radio, TV, and film from the University of Maryland.

Mr. Lampton has more than fifty non-fiction science books to his credit and nine works of fiction, including several science fiction novels for Doubleday and Laser Books. He currently lives outside Washington, D.C.